MW01489416

CARE OF THE FEET

Second Edition

William K. Ishmael, M.D.

Howard B. Shorbe, M.D.

J. B. LIPPINCOTT COMPANY Philadelphia
London   Mexico City   New York
St. Louis   São Paulo   Sydney

Your feet are among the most complex structures of your body. Each of your feet contains 26 bones, 19 muscles, and 107 ligaments (Fig. 1). Your foot is much more than a platform or support. It is actually a dynamic mechanism that must meet many challenges every day of your life. It must be flexible enough to adapt to the many kinds of surfaces on which you may walk. It must be strong enough to act as a lever and spring when you are walking. It must be sturdy enough to carry all of your weight every time you take a step, and to support you when you stand.

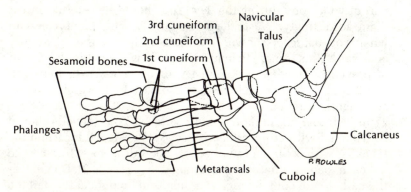

FIGURE 1.   Bones of the foot. (Christensen JB, Telford IR: Synopsis of Gross Anatomy, 4th ed, p 255. Philadelphia, Harper & Row, 1982)

If you are an average person, you walk approximately 8 miles every day, and many people have jobs requiring them to be on their feet for hours at a time. Under stresses like these, it is not surprising that almost everyone's feet give them trouble at some time during their life. This booklet will show you how to avoid having trouble with your feet and what you can do about trouble if you have it.

CARE OF HEALTHY FEET

"An ounce of prevention is worth a pound of cure."

This old saying can certainly apply to your feet. A normal foot is very strong and durable and will certainly take a lot of punishment before it will begin to hurt. However, why not do what you can to take care of your feet and ease the wear-and-tear they have to take? They will serve you better if you do, because pain in your feet can affect everything you do every day.

Here are some tips on how to take care of healthy feet:

1. *Keep your feet clean.* Your feet are probably the hardest working part of your body during the day. You should be careful to treat them accordingly. Wash them thoroughly with plenty of soap when you bathe or shower, and be sure to dry them carefully afterward. This is more than just simple hygiene—it is also a kind of preventive medicine. Keeping your feet clean will help you avoid problems such as itching or athlete's foot, which you can get even if you are not an athlete.

2. *Trim your toenails carefully and regularly.* Your toenails should be trimmed with clippers or with scissors designed for trimming toenails, which can be found at any good drugstore. It is best to cut each toenail square, that is, straight across (Fig. 2). Do not tear the nail, do not cut too much at a time, and do not cut the nail too short. File off any rough edges or slivers, which may tear later.

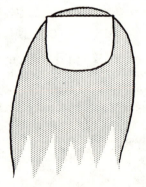

FIGURE 2. The nail is cut square (straight across) and, at the edges, extends past the skin of the toe.

Trim your toenails regularly—about every two weeks for most people. This is the best way to prevent ingrown toenail.

3. *Wear clean, good socks that fit.* Your socks or stockings are important, and you should wear a clean pair every day. Your socks or stockings should fit you as well as your shoes do. They should not feel "tight" or uncomfortable on your feet, nor should they wrinkle or feel too large or loose. Throw away or repair socks that develop holes, and do not wear socks that have worn thin on the bottom. Good, well-fitting socks will help you to avoid blisters and calluses.

You may want to wear extra-thick socks in cold weather or during strenuous activity such as hiking or running. If you do, be sure that your shoes or boots are large enough to accommodate the extra thickness. You may develop blisters if the extra-thick socks make your shoes or boots too tight.

4. *Wear good shoes that fit you well.* Wearing good shoes that fit you well is the most important thing that you can do to take care of your feet. Plain common sense is the best way for you to decide what shoes you should wear. Your own comfort as you perform your daily tasks is the best indicator of whether your shoes are good for your feet or not, and no one can be a better judge of this than you. If your feet do not hurt you and do not become unusually tired, then your shoes are probably all right. However, any shoe that makes your feet "tired," makes your feet hurt, or gives you any other discomfort, is wrong for you and should not be worn.

Figure 3 shows the parts of a practical, "ideal" shoe.

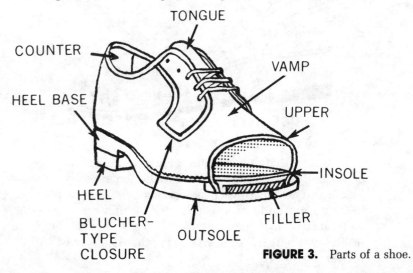

FIGURE 3. Parts of a shoe.

Here are some tips for choosing a well-fitting shoe:

For Women: The heel of your shoe should be from $\frac{3}{8}$ inch to $1\frac{1}{2}$ inches high. Ideally, your shoe's heel should be as wide as the heel of your foot. The narrower your shoe's heel, the less stability your foot will have. (With a very narrow heel, you may feel as if you are walking on ice skates!) At the minimum, the bottom of the heel of your shoe should be *at least half* as wide as the heel of your foot. If you are used to walking barefoot or in heel-less slippers, you may be comfortable in "flats." A shoe with a wedge heel is inexpensive and will give you excellent arch support.

Be sure that the traction surface of the heel—the part that strikes the ground—is made of a shock-absorbent, non-slip material.

When trying on a shoe, make sure that the heel cup fits the heel of your foot snugly. The cup should support your inner ankle and should be soft-lined. A blucher-type lacing as shown in the illustration of the "ideal" shoe (Fig. 3) will help to adjust the shoe and support the ankle. In a shoe without lacing, such as the shoe with a wedge heel shown in Figure 4, an adjustable heel strap serves the same purpose, but not as well.

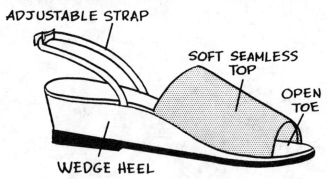

FIGURE 4. Woman's shoe with a wedge heel.

Make sure that the toe of the shoe does not create pressure or discomfort. It should conform to the general shape of your foot. If you are wearing a heel high enough to cause your foot to slide down and forward, a pointed toe may create pressure and thus may lead to or aggravate corns, soft corns, bunions, or ingrown nails. A shoe with a toe that is too tight will do the same.

You should check the top of the shoe carefully—it should be seamless and made of a soft material. When trying the shoe on, be sure that the "upper" (front) part of the shoe does not constrict or cause pressure across the top of your foot or your instep. Check that the "vamp" does not crease or wrinkle across the top of your foot. If you have unusually high arches, or if you wear inlays in your shoes, you must be particularly careful in checking the tightness of the vamp part of your shoe. You can have a shoe repairman stretch the vamp to form a "dome" before you wear new shoes.

Look very closely at the sole of the shoe, for that is its most important part. Its traction surface should be strong, firm, and made of a non-slip material. Look inside the shoe also. If you have corns or bunions, or other tender irregularities on your feet, you will want the inner sole of your shoe to be made of an impressionable material such as ground cork and rubber, or polyurethane foam. These materials will conform to the contour of your individual foot. "Pockets" will form to absorb the irregularities, thus lessening rubbing and discomfort.

For Men: If you have an average foot, you will probably not have much trouble with most men's shoes. However, it is still important to choose your shoes carefully, especially if you are heavier than the average man, or if you spend many hours on your feet.

The heel of your shoe should be at least as wide—or wider—than the heel of your own foot, and it should be approximately $\frac{7}{8}$ inch high.

Be sure that the traction surface of the heel—the part that strikes the ground—is made of a shock-absorbent, non-slip material.

When trying on a shoe, make sure that the heel cup fits the heel of your foot snugly. The cup should support your inner ankle and should be soft-lined.

Make sure that the toe of the shoe does not create pressure or discomfort. It should conform to the general shape of your foot. A pointed toe, or a toe that is too tight, may lead to or aggravate corns, soft corns, bunions, or ingrown nails.

You should check the top of the shoe carefully—it should be seamless and made of a soft material. When trying the shoe on, be sure that the "upper" (front) of the shoe does not constrict or cause pressure across the top of your foot or your instep. Check that the "vamp" does not crease or wrinkle across the top of your foot. If you have unusually high arches, or if you wear inlays in your shoes, you must be particularly careful in checking the tightness of the vamp part of your shoe. You can have a shoe repairman stretch the vamp to form a "dome" before you wear new shoes.

You should look very closely at the sole of the shoe, especially if you are a heavy man. Its traction surface should be strong, firm, and made of a non-slip material. Look inside the shoe also. If you have corns or bunions, or other tender irregularities on your feet, you will want the inner sole of your shoe to be made of an impressionable material such as ground cork and rubber, or polyurethane foam. These materials will conform to the contour of your individual foot. "Pockets" will form to absorb the irregularities, thus lessening rubbing and discomfort.

Work Shoes and Athletic Shoes: Shoes worn by either men or women in strenuous jobs or in active sports activities must be chosen with special care. If you work in industry or construction, *always* wear a shoe or boot designed for maximum safety and strength. As with ordinary shoes, common sense in choosing your work shoes will be your best guide.

Special shoes have been designed for most active sports activities. Your feet need these shoes to stand up to the unusual exercise and strain and to avoid painful injuries. Wear the right shoe, carefully fitted, for your sport. If you are just starting out in a sport, go to a store that specializes in shoes for athletes, and get their advice before you buy.

Children's Shoes: You should choose your children's shoes the same way that you choose your own. Remember that almost all children are much more active than the average adult. Their shoes will take more wear-and-tear than yours do, and will need to be replaced more often. Remember also that you should replace your children's shoes *before* they outgrow them. Allowing your child to wear shoes that are too small can cause permanent damage to the feet.

Care of Your Shoes: Don't buy cheap shoes—they will be more likely to hurt your feet, and they will definitely wear out faster. Get good shoes, take care of them and make them last, and you will get more for your money.

Try to have more than one pair of good shoes, so that you can alternate them day to day. Shoes need at least one day to dry after one ordinary day's wear. It is a good idea to insert shoe trees when the shoes are not being worn, especially if the shoes are wet. These will maintain the shape and fit of your shoes, and will prevent shrinking or curling up of the toes.

Break-in new shoes carefully and slowly. New shoes need time to adjust to your feet, and your feet need time to adjust to new shoes. Get waterproofing and polish, and apply them regularly to make your shoes last longer. They will look better too!

COMMON CAUSES OF FOOT PAIN AND WHAT TO DO ABOUT THEM

FATIGUE AND STRAIN

Tiredness in the foot and foot strain are common problems, especially among middle-aged and elderly people, and among people whose jobs require standing for long periods. Tiredness is the reaction of the muscles of your feet to too much exertion or work. At first, it is felt as a general aching or fatigue of the feet. If your feet are not rested, the pain will progress to aching under the arches, aching in your calves when you walk, swelling, and stiffness.

When this happens, your natural desire will be to get off your feet and rest them, and that is the best natural remedy. Soaking in warm water will help. Stay off your feet the next day if you can. If you must walk or stand, wear a different pair of shoes to help ease the strain. Usually, a day or two of rest will be enough.

If the muscles of your feet are too weak, however, strain and swelling can become a chronic condition. The toes may not be strong enough to remain properly straight during walking, so that they curl and rub against the uppers of your shoes, causing painful corns and calluses. Feet can stiffen and become painful, which can lead to persistent pain and aching in the calves.

You will need to see your physician if you develop such persistent pain. You may need to limit your activity for a time. The physician may suggest metatarsal pads (see Fig. 6) or arch supports for your shoes, to help relieve stress during standing and walking. Your physician may also suggest exercises to strengthen your feet (see "Exercises for the Feet" on p. 25).

BLISTERS, CALLUSES, CORNS, AND WARTS

Blisters, calluses, corns, and warts are all very common, and they all come from the same cause: pressure or friction. If you develop one of these conditions, it means that your shoes are not properly fitted to your feet and are causing unusual pressure or friction. The painful area on your foot is your foot's reaction to this pressure or friction. Changing to a better kind of shoe is the first thing to consider in relieving this pressure.

However, if your feet are of a slightly unusual shape, you may develop these problems even if you have chosen your shoes very carefully. And once a callus, wart, or corn has formed, it becomes self-perpetuating. It receives even more pressure and friction by rubbing itself against your shoe, and then becomes even more painful.

The way to treat such a problem is to eliminate the pressure that caused it in the first place. If your shoes are already the best you can find, then you will need to modify them in some manner. Merely stretching the top of the shoe to raise a dome over the area of a tender corn or callus will often relieve the pressure enough for it to heal.

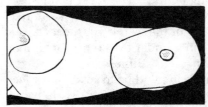

FIGURE 5. Pads to reduce pressure.

For mild corns or warts, a notched oval pad cut from adhesive felt, foam rubber, or polyurethane foam and placed in the shoe may help relieve the pressure (Figs. 5 and 6). Ready-to-use inlays may be

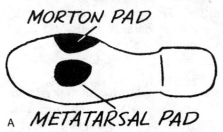

MORTON PAD

A   METATARSAL PAD

FIGURE 6. (A) Morton pad and metatarsal pad (continued on next page).

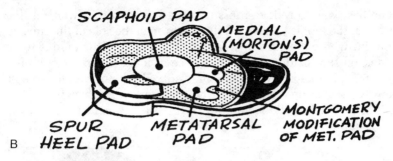

SCAPHOID PAD
MEDIAL (MORTON'S) PAD
MONTGOMERY MODIFICATION OF MET. PAD
SPUR HEEL PAD
METATARSAL PAD

B

FIGURE 6 (*continued*). (*B*) Various pads and inlays that may be used to reduce pressure on tender corns and calluses.

placed under the insole of the shoe (Fig. 7). It is possible to place such pads yourself, but it is best to see an orthotist or shoe repairman, to be sure that it is done properly.

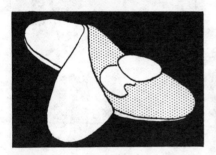
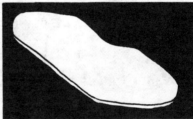

FIGURE 7. Inlays placed under insole to reduce pressure.

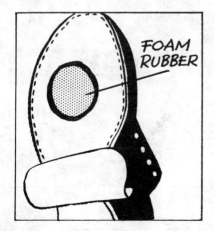

FOAM RUBBER

FIGURE 8. Hole cut through sole of shoe to avoid pressure on large plantar wart or callus.

The best way to relieve pressure on a larger corn or wart on the bottom of the foot is to have a hole cut through the sole of the shoe at the point where the corn or wart projects (Fig. 8). This hole is then padded on the inside with a thin piece of foam rubber or polyurethane foam before a new outer sole is affixed. The new outer sole is made thicker under the ball of the foot and thinner in front and behind, so that in walking your foot will "roll" over the painful area. This is called a rocker bar (Fig. 9).

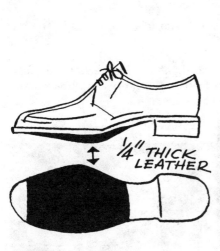

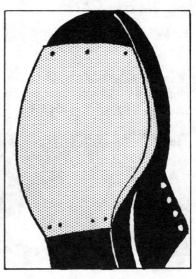

FIGURE 9. Rocker bar.

The metatarsal bar is a similar but simpler device for less painful corns or warts (Fig. 10). It is a piece of leather $\frac{1}{4}$ inch thick that is

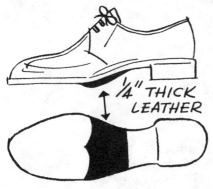

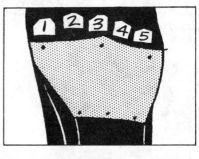

FIGURE 10. Metatarsal bar.

placed on the outer sole just behind the ball of the foot. Needless to say, any work of this kind must be done by an experienced orthotist or shoe repairman.

To immediately care for a corn or callus, you should soak your feet in warm, soapy water and then carefully rub them with a clean towel. You should not attempt to cut the corn or callus yourself. If it is severe enough to need cutting, then you should seek expert trimming from a podiatrist.

INGROWN TOENAIL

Ingrown toenail is a common and painful problem that most often affects the great (big) toe at the inner margin of the nail. An ingrown toenail curls inward into the skin, causing irritation and often infection. If infection is present, you should see your doctor immediately.

Shoes that are too narrow or too short and tight are usually the cause of an ingrown toenail. If you have a tendency to develop an ingrown toenail, you should take special care to trim your toenails properly, as shown in Figure 2.

Here are suggestions for temporary relief of pain caused by an ingrown toenail:

1. Thin the center of the nail by filing to relieve pressure on the edges (Fig. 11).

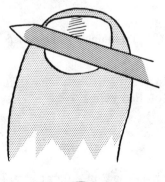

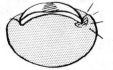

FIGURE 11. Thinning the nail in the center by filing reduces pressure at the edges.

2. If the nail is embedded, try wedging a fluff of cotton under the nail for temporary relief (Fig. 12).

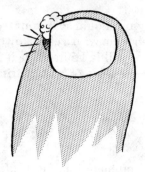

FIGURE 12.   Fluff of cotton wedged under the nail.

3. Or, trim the nail diagonally to its very edge, as shown in Figure 13.

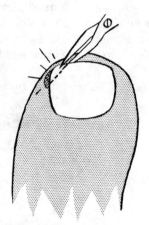

FIGURE 13.   Trimming the nail diagonally.

Remember, do not rely on these home treatments for a persistently painful toenail, or if infection is present. See your doctor.

ATHLETE'S FOOT

Athlete's foot is a fungus infection. It is caused by a damp, humid environment and by sweaty socks, which provide a good environment for the spread of fungus.

Usually you can prevent athlete's foot by washing your feet every day and drying them well, especially between the smaller toes. You should change your socks every day. For athletic activity, or other exertion that makes your feet sweat, you should be sure to wear properly ventilated shoes. If the weather is hot, or if your feet perspire excessively, you may want to use a foot powder. Cotton placed between the smaller toes will help keep those areas dry during athletic activity.

If you do develop a fungus infection, you may want to try a commercial preparation. However, if the infection persists, you should see your doctor.

FLAT FEET

Flat feet—or the lack of a well-developed muscular support to the arch of the foot—is a common condition. About one-third of adults have flat feet.

Usually, flat feet will cause only some awkwardness in walking and a tendency for the feet and calves to become tired and strained. You may wear out your shoes more quickly than most people do and you must be especially careful in choosing your shoes. If flat feet cause you severe fatigue or pain, you should see your doctor. He may suggest strengthening exercises for your feet (see "Exercises for the Feet" elsewhere in this booklet) or modifications to your shoes.

Most children are born with flat feet and develop normal arches by the age of 4 or 5. If your child has flat feet after this age, it is worth discussing the problem with your doctor because it is sometimes possible to correct flat feet in a growing child.

BUNION

A bunion (or "hallux valgus") is a very common deformity of the foot. It is not caused by your shoes, but your shoes can make a bunion very painful.

If your bunion is not too painful, you can "live with" it by being very careful to choose a shoe that conforms to the shape of your foot. You may also be helped by this exercise: Stretch the big toe longer, then pull it into a straight line. Maintain this position by pulling for several minutes.

A bunion can be cured only by an operation, and you should have this done if pain is serious or if you cannot find shoes to fit.

If your bunion joint becomes inflamed, you should see your doctor—it may suggest gout or arthritis.

HAMMERTOE

Hammertoe is a condition in which the toes are drawn up towards the ball of the foot, forcing the ball of the foot down and the joint of the toe up. This means that too much pressure is placed on the top of the toes and the ball of the foot when you are walking. The condition often results in painful corns and calluses.

One way to relieve this pain is by using protective pads of polyurethane foam. These are crinkle-cut in an accordion-like manner and cut in strips $\frac{1}{2}$ inch wide, $\frac{1}{4}$ inch thick, and 10 inches long. The strips can be looped comfortably between the toes or they can be placed as "buttress" pads under and over the toes (Fig. 14).

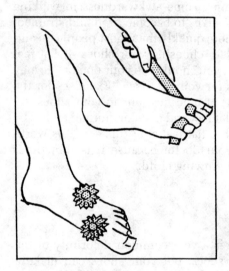

FIGURE 14. Use of crinkle-cut polyurethane foam (Ogden's Toeettes).

Wear open sandals or open-toe shoes whenever possible. Inlays may help when placed in properly fitted shoes.

Hammertoe can be relieved by these exercises:

- Stretch the affected toes longer, then flex them downward. Hold the toes in this stretched, flexed position for 3 to 5 minutes. This will stretch the tendons that pull the toes upward.
- Simply flex the toes downward 10 to 20 times.

- Walking on inlays in properly fitted shoes will help you maintain your toes in a flexed position, preventing the cocked-up position of the hammertoe.

If hammertoe gives you progressive and persistent trouble, you should have the problem corrected by an operation.

TAILOR'S BUNION

Tailor's bunion is a painful swelling of the joint at the base of the little toe. It is usually caused by pressure on the outer part of the joint.

You can relieve the pressure by wearing a doughnut-shaped pad over the joint in a properly fitted shoe. Also, having a dome stretched in the side of the shoe over the bunion will help to relieve the pressure.

If the joint becomes enlarged, it may be due to a disease, such as arthritis, or to injury. If the enlargement becomes severe, you should see your doctor for medical treatment or surgical correction.

CLAWFOOT

A clawfoot is a foot with a fixed, unusually high arch. Hammertoe or clawtoe can occur with clawfoot.

Clawfoot, also known as *pes cavus*, can be caused by any of several serious neurological or muscular diseases. Usually it appears in childhood, often by the time a child is 4 years old.

A child with clawfoot will have difficulty walking or running. This is a serious condition, and if you think your child may have clawfoot, an examination should be performed by your doctor.

Many people with clawfoot need custom-made shoes. People with clawfoot require special foot care throughout their lives.

MORTON'S TOE

The symptoms of Morton's toe are severe burning and cramp-like pain between the third and fourth toes. The pain is caused by compression of the nerve during standing or walking. Often the pain comes in spasms. Usually the condition results from too-tight shoes or from constantly wearing high-heeled shoes.

The attacks of pain can be relieved by getting off your feet and removing your shoes.

Often, Morton's toe can be controlled by wearing less constrictive, better designed shoes. Also, wearing a soft insole in the shoe may reduce pressure on the nerve.

If the problem continues, an operation may be needed.

SOFT CORN

A soft corn is a painful, soft nodule between two toes. It is caused by pressure in the area, usually because of a bony prominence or spur on the opposing toe or under the corn. Shoes that are too narrow can aggravate the problem.

The constant moisture between the toes keeps the soft corn from becoming hard like an ordinary pressure corn. A soft corn may become infected and is thus a serious problem.

Wider shoes can give some relief from a soft corn. You can also try wearing a protective pad between the toes to prevent the bony prominences from rubbing together. Lamb's wool or polyurethane foam can be used as padding.

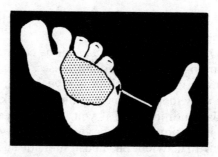

FIGURE 15. Use of padding for soft corn.

Or you can wear a thin felt pad that has been trimmed into a shape like that of a duck's head (Fig. 15). Place the round portion under the ball of the foot and then pull the long, bill-like strip up between the adjacent toes to hold them apart. This will relieve pressure on the corn.

If the corn persists or becomes infected, surgical removal of the bony spur may be necessary.

PAINFUL HEELS

Your heels may be painful for many reasons. The most common cause of heel pain is a badly fitted shoe that causes a blister on the back of the heel.

Pain can also be caused by an injury that strains the attachment of the Achilles tendon (heel cord) to the heel bone. You should treat such a strain as you would a sprained ankle: rest the area for 2 or 3 weeks until it heals.

You may also have pain on the weight-bearing part (the sole) of the heel. Ligaments supporting the arch of your foot are attached here, and if they are strained or inflamed, they can become painful. A bony spur may develop because of the stress. Arthritis may also be a cause of pain in this area, making it very tender over long periods of time, so that it feels like a childhood stone bruise.

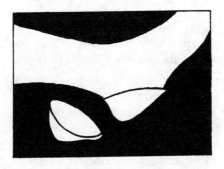

FIGURE 16. Heel pad or "jumper's cup" made of translucent plastic.

You can reduce heel pain by wearing a heel pad or "jumper's cup" (Fig. 16). This protects the heel from friction or pressure caused by your shoe, and will also cushion the heel if you have a bony spur or bursitis in the heel. Protective padding (spur heel pad) as shown in Figures 5 and 6 may also help.

Bursitis is indicated by a painful mass on the back of the heel. A chronically enlarged or acutely inflamed mass is a matter for your doctor, because it may indicate gout or some other form of arthritis. Occasionally, surgery may be needed to remove the mass.

MEDICAL CONDITIONS
THAT MAY AFFECT THE FEET

No one part of your body can be considered completely separate from the rest, and your feet are no exception. There are a number of diseases that are not diseases of the feet themselves, yet which can affect the feet and make it necessary for you to take special care of your feet. Here are some common disorders that often affect the feet, with suggestions for care.

DIABETES MELLITUS

Diabetes is a very common disorder involving the body's metabolism of sugar. If you have diabetes, your doctor has undoubtedly given you information and instructions for treatment. One of the results of diabetes can be poor circulation of blood to the feet, damage to the nerve supply, and lowered resistance to infection. For these reasons, you must be especially careful to keep your feet clean and to protect them from cuts, scrapes, blisters, or any other open wounds.

Here are some rules for foot care if you have diabetes:

1. Choose your shoes carefully, according to the suggestions earlier in this booklet. When you buy new shoes, break them in slowly.
2. Wear clean socks or stockings every day. Be sure that they fit properly, and do not let them wrinkle inside your shoes.
3. Keep your feet very clean. You should wash them daily with mild soap and water. Do not use water that is too hot. Do not add medicinals such as epsom salts.
4. Do not use hot water bottles or a heating pad for your feet. A burn could result in an ulcer.
5. Have someone else trim your toenails.
6. Do not trim corns or calluses yourself. If they are mild, soften them in warm, soapy water and carefully rub them off. Otherwise, see a podiatrist for trimming.
7. Do not wear circular garters or any other constrictive stocking that interferes with circulation.
8. If any sores or ulcers develop on your feet, tell your doctor at once.
9. If you injure your foot, do not apply adhesive tape to the skin and do not bandage the foot tightly. Avoid all strong liniments. Stay off the injured foot and keep it in an elevated position.

10. Do not wear metal arch supports.

11. Remember that tobacco may aggravate any circulatory problems.

12. Do not use commercial corn remedies or any sharp instruments on your feet. Do not walk barefoot or open blisters yourself.

REMEMBER: If you have diabetes, you should call your doctor immediately if any foot problems develop. With diabetes, any foot problem may be serious.

CIRCULATORY DISORDERS

The delivery of too little blood to the feet—poor circulation—may cause your feet to be painful. Frequent and painful muscle cramping or worsening pain that forces you to stop and rest may be symptoms of a circulatory disorder. If you have these symptoms, you should see your doctor. A circulatory disorder is a serious problem.

Varicose (enlarged) veins, heart disease, some kinds of kidney disease, and several other diseases can all cause swelling of the feet. If you have persistently swollen feet, you should see your doctor.

If you have any circulatory disorder, you should follow the same rules for foot care that are listed on page 20 for diabetes.

Do not confuse frequent, painful muscle cramping during exertion with occasional nighttime cramping ("Charley horse") or cramping of the feet at rest. An occasional "Charley horse" is painful, but it does not usually indicate a serious problem. See your doctor if exercise or walking regularly brings on cramping in your legs.

GOUT (GOUTY ARTHRITIS)

Gout is a form of arthritis that has a tendency to affect the feet. Gout is caused by abnormal levels of uric acid in the body and can produce extremely painful attacks of joint inflammation. Gout can affect any joint but by far the most common is the bunion joint of the big toe.

If you have gout, you are familiar with the symptoms of gradually increasing throbbing pain in the joint. Often an attack starts at night. After a few hours the joint becomes swollen, red, and very tender. Walking usually becomes impossible. If it is not treated, an attack will usually last for a week or two, after which the joint will return to normal.

If you have gout, it is very important that you avoid any injury or strain to the feet, because many joint attacks follow strain. It is essential that you wear properly fitted shoes at all times according to the guidelines given earlier in this booklet. It is also important that you keep your feet clean and avoid abrasions or cuts. Follow the suggestions for special foot care given for people with diabetes.

If you have an advanced case of gout, you may have developed lumps of chalky crystals called tophi in the tissues around the inflamed joint. Tophi may need to be removed surgically.

Having gout means that you will have to continue under your doctor's care for this disease all your life. No longer having painful attacks does *not* mean you are cured.

RHEUMATOID ARTHRITIS

If you have rheumatoid arthritis, you must follow the instructions of your doctor regarding foot care. Many people with this disease have foot trouble of some kind, ranging from a swollen joint or limp to actual deformity and crippling. You should protect your feet from strain and abuse, and follow whatever physical therapy or exercises may be recommended by your doctor.

NEUROLOGIC PROBLEMS

Disorders of the nervous system can affect the feet. Paralysis, numbness, oversensitivity, severe burning, muscle cramping, and serious weakness are all symptoms that may indicate a problem or disease of the nervous system. If you notice any of these symptoms in your feet, you should see your doctor.

Do not confuse minor twitches or aches with symptoms of neurologic problems. Usually a "restless leg" or aching feet simply indicate fatigue. You should not be concerned unless these symptoms continue after you have had plenty of rest.

FROSTBITE (FROZEN FOOT)

Frostbite, or a frozen foot, is always an emergency, especially if you have any circulatory disorder or other disease affecting the feet. Rewarm the affected foot by gentle rubbing with a warm hand. Emergency treatment involves immersing the frozen part in warm, but not hot, water. See your doctor immediately.

EXERCISES FOR THE FEET

The best exercise for your feet is walking properly in a good pair of shoes. "Proper" walking is walking with your toes pointed forward or turned in slightly, especially if you have flat feet or problems with sagging ankles. Walking with your toes turned in or out too much can contribute to foot strain and fatigue. You should try to walk as briskly and vigorously as you can.

On a long walk, relax occasionally if you can, and rest your feet. Remove your shoes and stretch and massage the joints of the feet.

If you have flat feet, sagging ankles, or similar problems, you may want or need to strengthen your feet with exercises specifically for them. Here are some suggestions:

- In a standing position, rise on tiptoe 5 to 10 times, and then walk 10 to 20 steps on tiptoe (Fig. 17). This will strengthen your

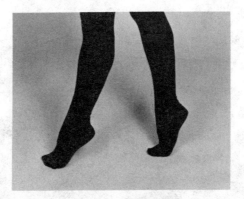

FIGURE 17.

calf muscles, heel cord, and muscles of the feet. Note that you should reduce or stop this exercise if it persistently causes increased morning stiffness. You will not be able to do this exercise if you have significant problems with your toes or the joints of your feet.

- In a standing position, turn your ankles outward, so that your body weight is borne on the other side of your feet (Fig. 18). Repeat this motion 5 to 10 times. Then walk 10 to 20 steps, continuing to bear your body weight on the outer sides of your feet. This exercise will help to strengthen ankles that sag in.

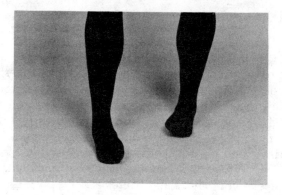

FIGURE 18.

- Remove your shoes and hold onto a table or chair to maintain your balance. Squat as low as possible, until your buttocks rest on your heels (Fig. 19). Keep your heels on the floor as long as you can. This exercise will stretch your heel cords (Achilles tendon), and it is especially good for women who wear high heels.

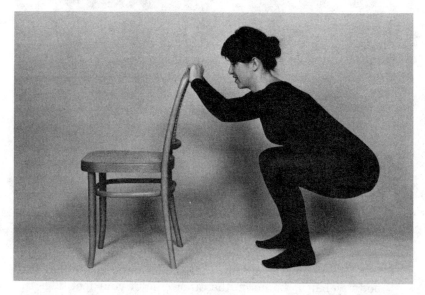

FIGURE 19.

- If your knees or hips are stiff and will not allow you to do the above stretching exercise, you can simply stand with the balls of your feet on a 1-inch high object, such as a book, and let your heels rest on the floor (Fig. 20). This will also stretch the Achilles tendon and other tendons, ligaments, and muscles on the backs of your legs.

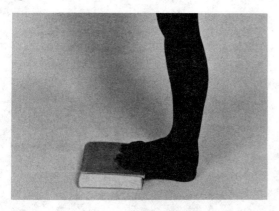

FIGURE 20.

- Another stretching exercise can be performed by lifting your feet and toes up and walking with all your weight carried on your heels (Fig. 21). While doing this, keep the balls of your feet lifted upward as much as possible. This will not only stretch your Achilles tendon but will also stretch the muscles on the tops of your feet and the fronts of your legs.

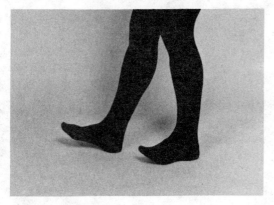

FIGURE 21.

Here is a program of exercises specifically designed to help people who have weak, chronically strained, and aching feet:

First, bathe your feet in two pans or buckets of water, one as hot and the other as cold as your feet can stand. Hold your feet in the hot water for 1 minute and hold them in the cold water for half a minute. Repeat this 5 times. Then dry your feet vigorously with a rough towel. Perform these exercises 6 times at first, working up to 12:

1. Sit on a chair with your feet on a towel. Keep your toes straight by pressing them against the towel with your fingers. Then try to bring your heels toward your toes, so that you slowly lift your arches (Fig. 22). Keep your knees together firmly.

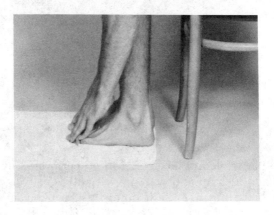

FIGURE 22.

2. Raise your toes while keeping all the rest of your feet firmly on the floor (Fig. 23).

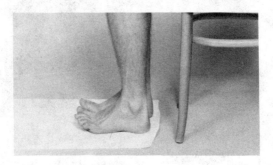

FIGURE 23.

3. Arch your feet and turn them in until the big toes and balls of the feet touch (Fig. 24). Keep your knees together and the outer borders of your feet on the floor throughout the exercise.

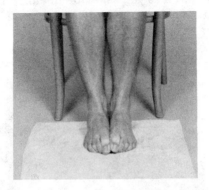

FIGURE 24.

4. Use your toes to claw the towel into a ball under your feet. Pick up a pencil or other graspable object with your toes (Fig. 25).

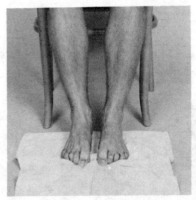

FIGURE 25.   A

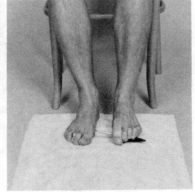

B

5. Put your foot on the chair so that the ball of the foot and your toes are extended just over the edge. Flex and extend your toes while using your fingers to resist the movements (Fig. 26). Then spread out your toes as far as you can without either flexing or extending them. If you cannot spread your big toe, move it with your fingers and then try to hold it in that position.

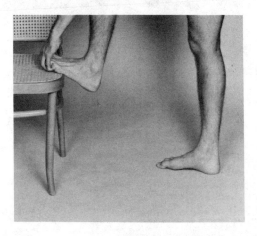

FIGURE 26.

6. Raise your heels as high as you can, while keeping your toes straight and the balls of your feet on the floor (Fig. 27).

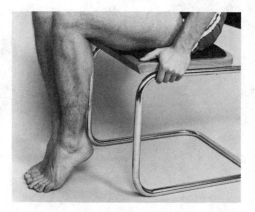

FIGURE 27.

After you have done these exercises two or three times a day for two weeks in a sitting position, you can do exercises 1, 2, 3, and 6 while standing. You should start again with 6 repetitions and work up to 12 repetitions.

IF YOU ARE THINKING ABOUT BECOMING A RUNNER

Running is wonderful exercise, but it does place a lot of extra strain and stress on your feet. Every time you run one mile, each foot strikes the ground about 800 times. If you weigh 150 pounds, that means that each of your feet receives 60 tons of impact each time you run a mile. Think of the impact your feet receive if you can run more than a mile! And all of this impact passes through your feet and is felt by your ankles, knees, hips, and back.

So you should pay special attention to your feet if you are going to run. Don't wear ordinary sneakers or tennis shoes for running. Go to a good athletic equipment store and get shoes designed for running. There are several chains of stores that specialize in shoes and running equipment, and you can usually receive expert advice in choosing shoes from the sales clerk.

Try the shoes on carefully while wearing the socks that you plan to run in. Make sure that the heel is wide enough to be comfortable but not loose. Make sure that your toes have plenty of room, but that your foot does not slide forward. The soles should be well-padded, with padding that is firm but not hard—there should be some "give." Test the flexibility of the shoe, especially at the ball of the foot. If the shoe seems hard for you to bend, or takes unusual effort as you push off with a stride, don't buy it.

After you have begun a program of running, it is important to pay attention to the condition of your feet, and to look for any early signs of trouble. Keep your toenails closely trimmed. Otherwise, when your toes strike the front of your shoes on impact, the nails will be damaged by the force so that they may turn black or even—eventually—fall off. Use sterile gauze to cover any small blisters that develop.

Pain in the heels can be due to a number of conditions, usually caused by too many repeated blows to the feet during running. Heel cups or other padding will usually relieve the problem and allow you to continue running. If the pain persists or worsens, you may need to rest until the injury heals, or see a podiatrist or your regular doctor.

Stress fractures can occur in the bones of the toes (or in the bones of the lower leg). They feel like bruised feet, or shin splints if they are in the leg. They are not usually serious, but you must reduce your running and get sufficient rest so that the stress fractures can heal. Do not try to ignore the pain. Running on a softer surface, rather than on pavement, may help to prevent recurrence.

Stretch your legs, back, stomach, and upper body thoroughly before you run—ideally, for about 10 minutes.

Finally, learn from experience—talk to experienced runners. And see your doctor if you have unexpected problems.

FOOT CARE FOR THE ELDERLY

It is not surprising that elderly people need to pay careful attention to their feet. Problems such as stiffness and sagging arches are common and natural after many years of strain and stress. The suggestions in this booklet regarding care of the feet and fitting of shoes are of special importance to you if you are elderly, because you are naturally prone to problems of the feet.

It is important to keep your feet clean at all times. Dirt left embedded in the folds of the skin can lead to scaling and shedding and even to inflammation (dermatitis), which can in turn lead to infection.

Be sure that your toenails are trimmed regularly and carefully. If you have difficulty reaching your toenails, or problems with your eyesight, have a family member, friend, or nurse help you.

Many older people have pain from calluses. If the calluses are not protected or removed, they can lead to pressure sores, which can become infected. If you develop calluses frequently, it is a good idea to see a podiatrist regularly.

Take special care to keep your feet warm and dry at all times. In wet or cold weather, wear thick socks and warm, waterproof boots or shoes. Be sure that your boots or shoes accommodate the extra-thick socks comfortably, and are not too tight or constricting.

NOTES